I Woke Up Fat!
31 Days of Clean Eating
...well, sipping really.

—

Drink your nutrients

Cecelia E. Fernandez

ISBN: 1497437466
ISBN 13: 9781497437463

My Vision

...is to write a 31-day guidebook with ideas and suggestions about smoothies. I know by now you must be thinking, *not another book about smoothies and juicing...somebody pass me a sandwich!*

I won't claim to know it all although at times I think I do. I am simply penning my ideas on how smoothies can be incorporated into our busy lives. I recently did a three-day food cleanse. We said good-bye to a very brutal winter and all its storms with names. Spring sprung but my body still felt trapped in the icebox called winter. I decided to renew my system on a cellular level by only sipping my nutrition.

I created my own cleanse in terms of smoothies that I love and puréed soups, basically putting my digestive system on vacation. I felt great and lost a few pounds in the process.

Smoothies are wonderful vehicles that transport your palate to destinations of intrigue or delight.

This book won't instruct you to use measures of this and measures of that. Instead, you are free to use the pictures as inspirational guides. This is not a diet book, but a change your food lifestyle guide.

Now let's blend to the betterment of our health.

I Woke Up Fat!
31 Days of Clean Eating
...well, sipping really.

—

Drink your nutrients

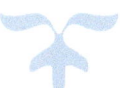

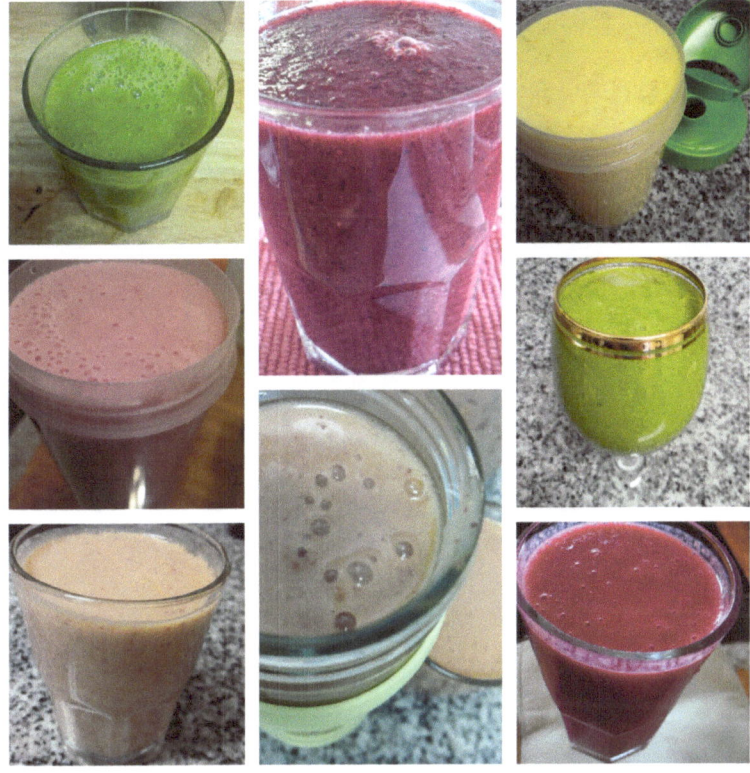

Acknowledgments

How do I thank thee? Let me count the ways.

1. To my darling husband, Claude, thank you for allowing me to sway you from your absolute disdain for vegetables. Yes, folks, he now makes his own avocado, tomato, celery, spinach, kale, lemon, and banana smoothie. We shall call this smoothie the Claudy ;-).

2. My dear sweet sister, Bronwyn, though we are separated by a vast body of water (she lives in South Africa), we are as close as can be. Thank you for being my shoulder to cry on and my ear when I just need to go on and on about smoothies and their endless health benefits.

3. The smoothie group of Sister-Friends who are always ready for a new and refreshing way to create magic with fruit and vegetables: Liesl, Sidonia, Wendy-Joy, Robyn-Lee, Tanya, Joy, and Caroline :-)

4. Thank you to the group of women who went from being my friends to my family: Khadija, Irina, Holli B, Lillian, and Amy Z.

5. MSM's teachers, thank you for embracing the smoothie basket.

6. Lastly, Bridie, my editor at large. Thank you for your wordy guidance. Thank you for assisting me with this mammoth project. Thank you for your willingness to food experiment with me. I am so blessed to have you as my friend, family, boss, and Rev.

Much love, care, and appreciation,
Cecelia
—xox—

Contents

MY STORY

Allow me to introduce myself. My name is Cecelia and I have been making smoothies for the greater part of twenty years. I was born and raised in Cape Town, South Africa, where most, if not all, of 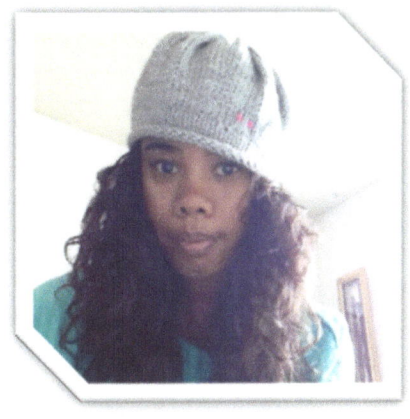 our meals were farm to table, ocean to table, or vineyard to glass☺. It was cheaper and frankly healthier to eat this way.

My passion for making smoothies is what drove me to pen this book. Smoothies——what an amazingly healthy, fast, and exciting way to get vital nutrients into our bodies.

The fervor for making smoothies kicked in when my mom passed away. That was when I realized my health must be important to me. I am responsible for this vessel called Cecelia's body.

I started reading books on nutrition, constantly talked to nutritionists and fitness trainers, and watched food documentaries. I made going back to good nutrition my mission in life. Most, if not all, of my friends can attest to the fact that I am always food or smoothie chatting, so much so that we now have a smoothie basket at work. We place random bits of fruit and vegetables in said basket and I make smoothies for the teachers. I have converted the "oh! I don't like vegetables" folks to now sip the greenest of green drinks.

I have adopted this very firm belief that food can be used as medicine. Allow nature to be your chemist. I work at the Montessori School of Manhattan, and the Montessori philosophy is to believe in the whole being, the wholeness of self. Respect yourself and others; grace and courtesy are key. So, you see my work life fits my personal life's philosophy. We need annual medical physicals for school, and I see it as a personal challenge to "pass" my blood tests. Silly, right? You get to make your "score" perfect.

Don't get me wrong I will take the drugs if I have pain beyond human comprehension :-). I am in excellent health and I intend on blending my way to greatness.

Thank you for reading my story.

—xox—

Tummy Wellness

INGREDIENTS

1 cup Pineapple	1 cup Mango	2 Tbsp. grated Ginger	¼ cup Aloe Vera Gel or Juice

I feel like a responsible adult when I drink this smoothie, knowing that I am taking care of my digestive health.

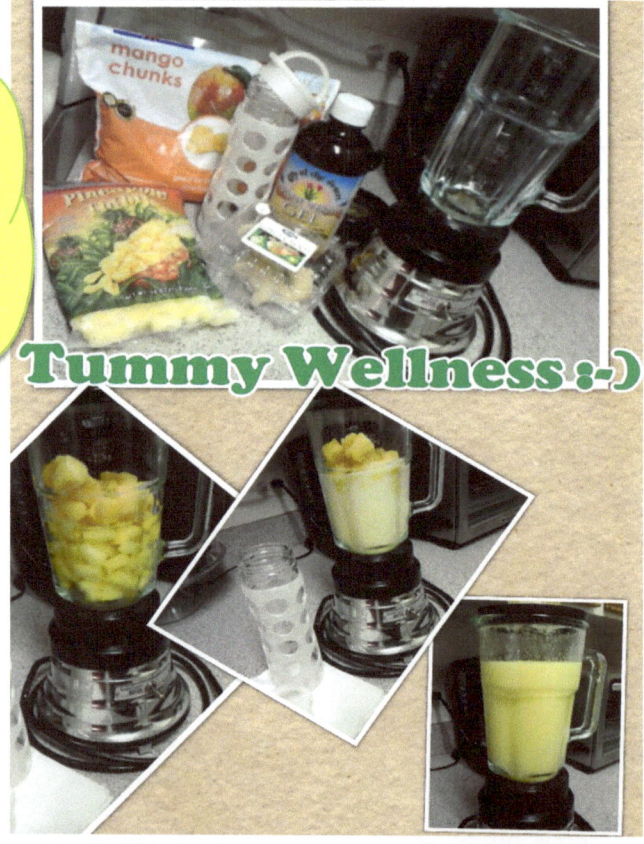

Tummy Wellness :-)

Notepad

My 30 Day Smoothie Guide

Day 1	Day 2	Day 3	Day 4	Day 5	NOTES
Flax Seeds	Hemp Seeds	Chia Seeds	Cacao Powder	Flax Seeds	
Kefir	Kefir	Silk - Coconut Milk	Almond Milk	Coconut Water	
Mango	Banana	Banana	Almond Butter	Spinach	
Kale	Pineapple	Peaches	Kale	Ginger	
Straw berries	Spinach	Mango	Banana	Green Apple	

Day 6	Day 7	Day 8	Day 9	Day 10
Flax Seeds	Chia Seeds	Hemp Seeds	Flax Seeds	Bee Pollen
Orange Bell Pepper	Almond Milk	Coconut Water	Water	Water
Orange	Almond Butter	Kale	Spinach	Carrot
Carrot	Kale	Banana	Mango	Straw berries
Coconut Oil	Blueberries	Spinach	Green Apple	Orange Bell Pepper
Mango	Banana	Celery	Lemon	Banana

Day 11	Day 12	Day 13	Day 14	Day 15
Flax Seeds	Chia Seeds	Hemp Seeds	Flax Seeds	Bee Pollen
Aloe Gel	Coconut Water	Coconut Water	Coconut w ater	Mint
Cucumber	Orange	Orange Bell Pepper	Banana	Banana
Parsley	Peaches	Mango	Spinach	Watermelon
Celery	Pineapple	Carrots	Almond Butter	Mixed Berries
Spinach	Banana	Lemon	Lemon	Ginger
Kale	Straw berries	Lemon zest	Lemon zest	Peaches
Banana	Cayenne Pepper	Ginger	Raspberries	

Day 16	Day 17	Day 18	Day 19	Day 20
Flax Seeds	Chia Seeds	Flax Seeds	Hemp Seeds	Flax Seeds
Coconut Water	Silk - Coconut Milk	Almond milk	Coconut w ater	Silk - Coconut Milk
Blueberries	Mango	Overnight soaked oats	Kale	Pineapple
Mango	Overnight soaked oats	Banana	Parsley	Melon (any kind)
Kale, Avocado	Apricots x2	Spinach	Spinach	Carrot
Lemon	Kale	Cinnamon	Celery	Straw berries
Lemon zest	Pineapple	Honey (if you need)	Grapefruit	Lemon
Cayenne Pepper		Almond Butter	Lemon, Orange	Lemon zest

Day 21	Day 22	Day 23	Day 24	Day 25
Flax Seeds	Hemp Seeds	Chia Seeds	Hemp Seeds	Chia Seeds
Silk - Coconut Milk	Green Tea (cooled)	Almond milk	Silk - Coconut Milk	Kefir
Banana	Soy milk (a splash)	Overnight soaked oats	Ginger	Flaxseed
Nutella	Banana	Blueberries	Kale	Orange
Straw berries	Melon	Peaches	Pineapple	Peaches
Peaches	Peaches	Almond milk	Peaches	Grapefruit
Celery		Celery	Celery	Carrot

Day 26	Day 27	Day 28	Day 29	Day 30
Hemp Seeds	Flax Seeds	Chia Seeds	Flax Seeds	Hemp Seeds
Almond Milk	Coconut Water	Water	Coconut Water	Almond Milk
Spinach	Tomato	Kefir	Grapefruit	Almond Butter
Parsley	Avocado	Steamed Beets	Orange	Straw berries
Banana	Lemon	Straw berries	Lemon	Cherries
Pear	Lemon zest	Raspberries	Lemon zest	Banana
Kale	Mango	Banana	Avocado	Kale
Peaches	Celery	Mango	Parsley	Pear
Lemon	Ginger	Pear	Cayenne Pepper	

SHOPPING LIST

CATEGORY	ITEMS			
1. THE LIQUIDS	Water	Coconut Water	Kefir	Aloe Gel/Juice
	Almond Milk	Coconut Milk	Soy Milk	Coconut Milk
2. THE SEEDS	Chia Seeds	Flaxseed	Hemp Seeds	Bee Pollen
3. THE FREEZER FILLERS	Mango	Strawberries	Mixed Berries	Blueberries
	Peaches	Cherries	Pineapple	Grapes (freeze fresh ones
4. THE CITRUS	Lemons	Grapefruit	Oranges	Limes
5. THE GREENS	Spinach	Kale	Celery	Parsley
6. THE BUTTERS	Almond Butter	Peanut Butter	Soy Nut Butter	Sunflower Butter	Nutella
7. THE FILL-ME-UP CREW	Oats	Banana	Apples	Orange Bell Peppers
8. THE FLAVOR AGENTS	Turmeric	Cinnamon	Honey/ Agave	Cayenne Pepper
NOTES				

THE TOOLS

- A good blender
- Zip-top baggies or containers
- A spill-proof bottle to take along with you as you go about your day

THE BASICS

- You do not have to stick to the above list; it is merely a guide.
- Buy the ingredients that you like to eat. If you enjoy eating it, then you will enjoy sipping it.
- I add lemon, lemon juice, and lemon zest to most of my smoothies. I find it brightens the color and perks up the flavor.
- Water will be your best friend. Drink it up and use some to thin your smoothies.
- Think of a smoothie as you would your wardrobe. You mix and match your outfits, so mix and match your smoothies. Once you have the basic pieces in your closet, the possibilities become endless. Dress your palate in different colors and flavor combinations!
- Use the notepads provided to create your own smoothies.

Breakfast with Nanna

INGREDIENTS

1 cup Coconut Milk	½ cup cooked Oats	1 Tbsp. Sunflower Seed Butter	1 tsp. Cinnamon	Day 1
Place all ingredients in blender. Blend until desired consistency.				

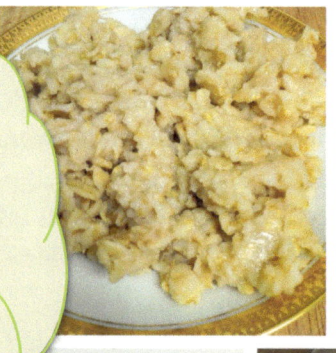
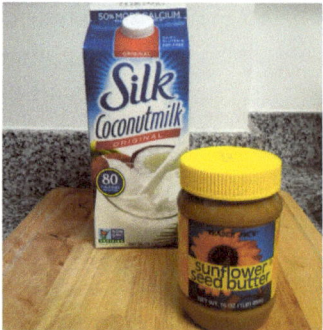

This smoothie is creamy, light, and delicious. Feel free to thin the mix with a splash of water.

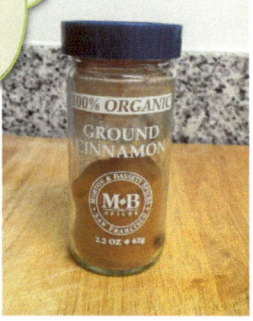
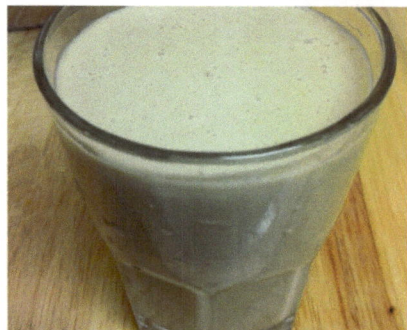

Notepad

From Daytime to Nighttime

INGREDIENTS

¼ cup Water	1 cup Carrots	2 cups Pineapple	4–6 Mint leaves	Day 2
1 Grapefruit	1 Banana	Place all ingredients in blender. Blend until desired consistency.		

This smoothie is not just for the start to your day. Add a shot or two of light Rum and Happy Hour is here!!

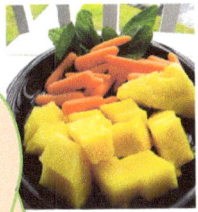
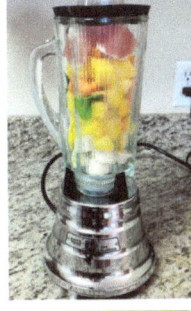
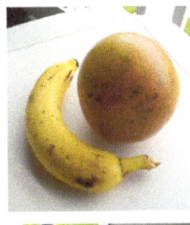
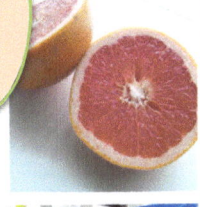
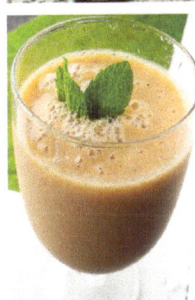
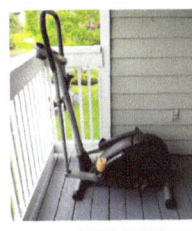
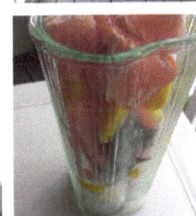

Notepad

Go Green

INGREDIENTS

1 cup fresh squeezed Orange Juice	½ cup fresh squeezed Lemon Juice	2 cups Spinach	3 sprigs Parsley	1 Banana	*Day* 3
1 Grapefruit	1 cup Pineapple	Place all ingredients in blender. Blend until desired consistency.			

This is a great make-ahead smoothie.

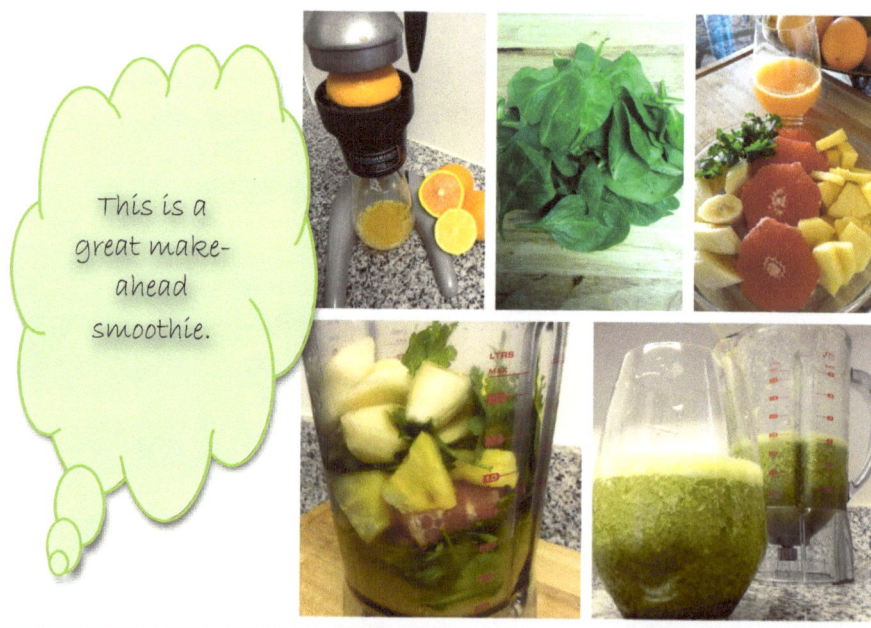

Notepad

A Little Nutty

INGREDIENTS

1 cup Almond Milk	1 Tbsp. Ground Flaxseed	2 cups Strawberries	4–6 Basil leaves	Day 4
1 cup Mango	½ Lemon	Place all ingredients in blender. Blend until desired consistency.		

Blend on low speed. Add less Almond Milk and this smoothie becomes a slushie ☺

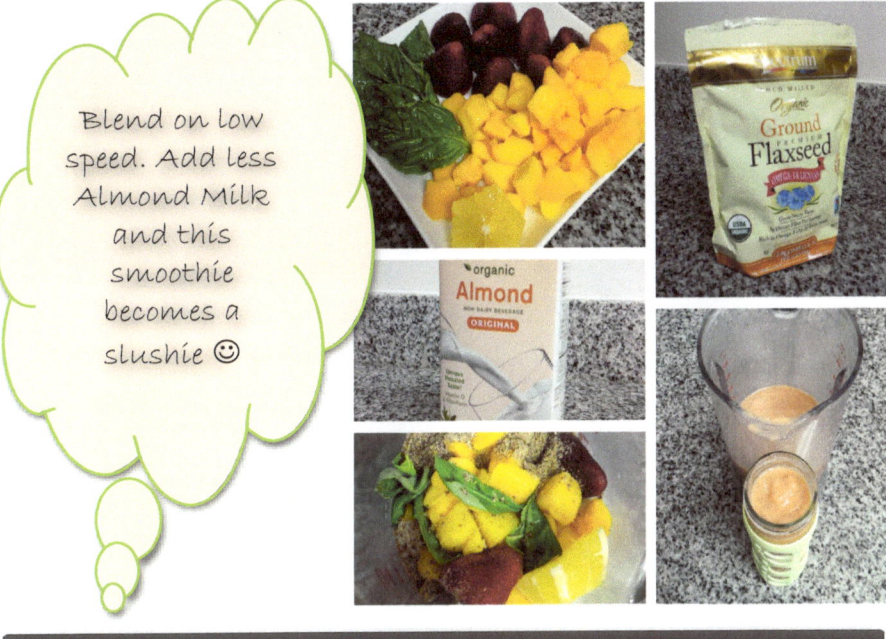

Notepad

Breakfast + Lunch = Brunch Time

INGREDIENTS

1 cup Coconut Milk	1 Tbsp. Chia Seeds	1 cup Oats soaked overnight	½ cup Mango	3 dried Apricots	Day 5
1 Banana	Place all ingredients in blender. Blend until desired consistency.				

The melting ice automatically thins this smoothie as well as keeps it cold.

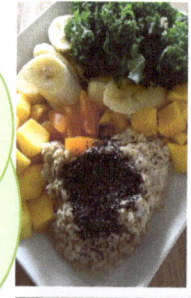
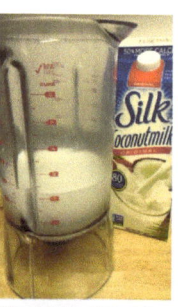
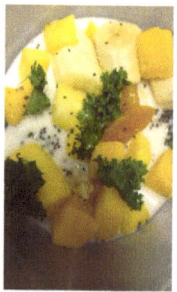
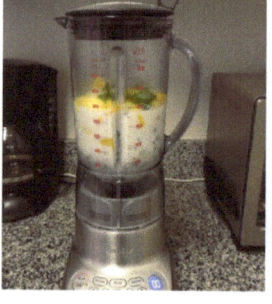
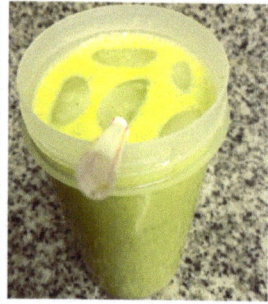

Notepad

Spa-Gua

INGREDIENTS

1 cup Coconut Water	1 Tbsp. Hemp Seeds	4–6 Mint leaves	1 Grapefruit	**Day 6**
½ Lemon	1 Orange	Place all ingredients in blender. Blend until desired consistency.		

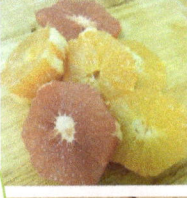
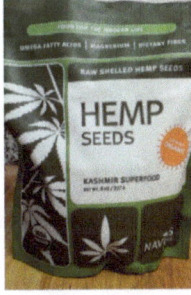
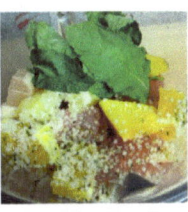
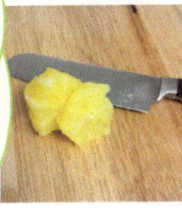
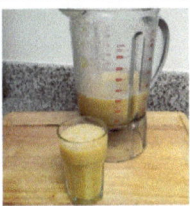

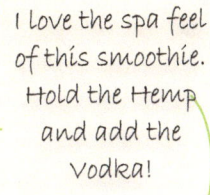

I love the spa feel of this smoothie. Hold the Hemp and add the Vodka!

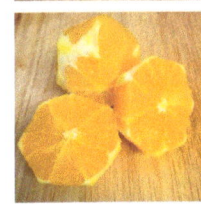
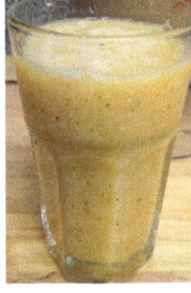
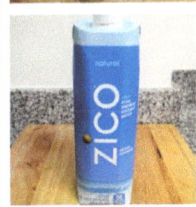

Notepad

Springtime in a Blender

INGREDIENTS

¼ cup Water	1 Tbsp. Chia Seeds	2 cups Watermelon	1 cup Mango	4–6 Basil leaves	Day 7
Place all ingredients in blender. Blend until desired consistency.					

The Basil gives this smoothie a subtle floral taste. I enjoy the freshness of this drink.

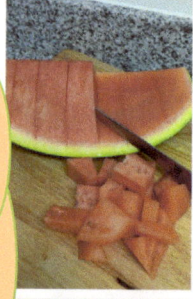
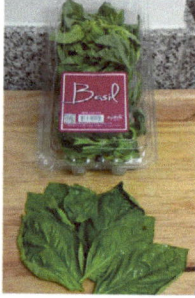
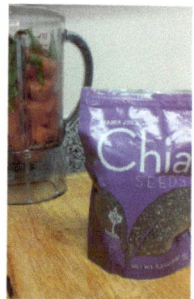
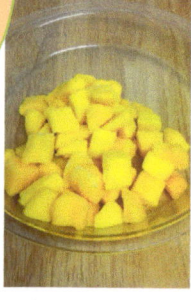
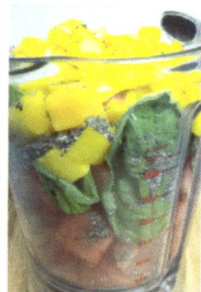
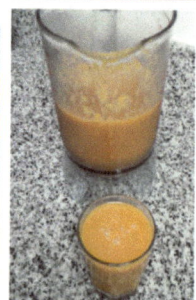

Notepad

Detox-a-Liscious

INGREDIENTS

1 cup Coconut Water	1 Tbsp. Hemp Seeds	2 large Kale leaves	2 cups Spinach	3 Parsley sprigs	Day 8
2 Celery stalks	1 Grapefruit	½ Lemon	1 Orange	Place all ingredients in blender. Blend until desired consistency.	

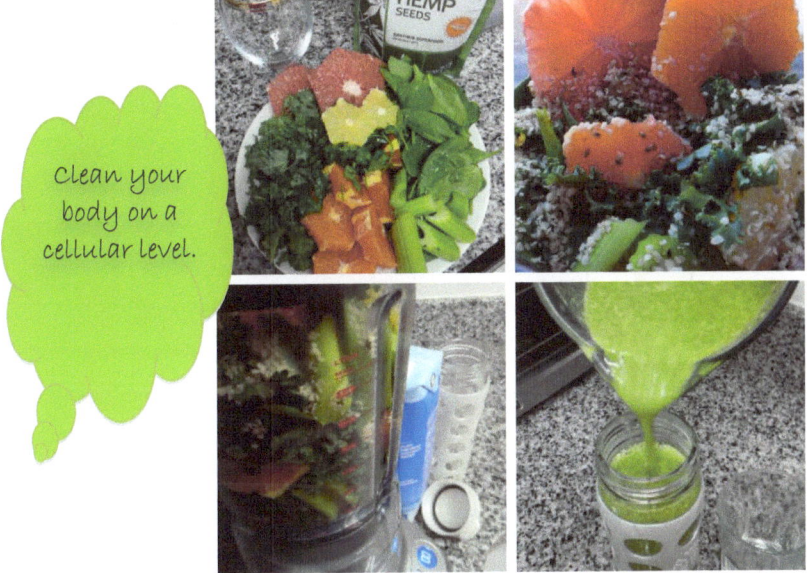

Clean your body on a cellular level.

Notepad

Florida Sun

INGREDIENTS

1 cup Coconut Milk	1 Tbsp. Hemp Seeds	1 cup Mango	½ Yellow Bell Pepper	1 cup Pineapple	**Day 9**
1 Banana	2 Celery stalks	Place all ingredients in blender. Blend until desired consistency.			

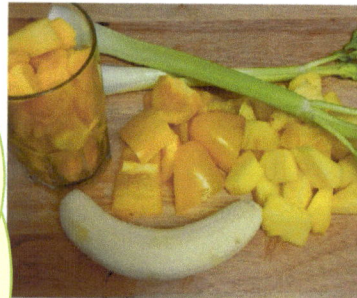
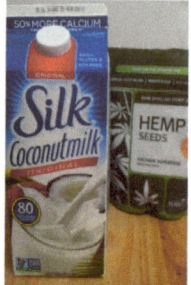

The vibrant soul-soothing yellow of this smoothie reminds me of Florida's sunny days.

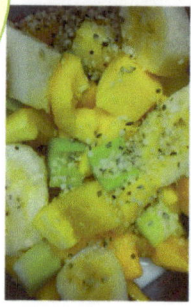
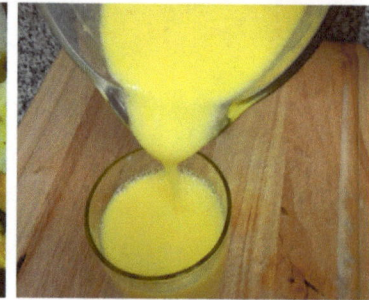

Notepad

Let's Get Our Probiotic On

INGREDIENTS

½ cup Kefir	1 Tbsp. Chia Seeds	2 cups Strawberries	1 Tomato	1 Banana	Day 10
¼ cup Water	Place all ingredients in blender. Blend until desired consistency.				

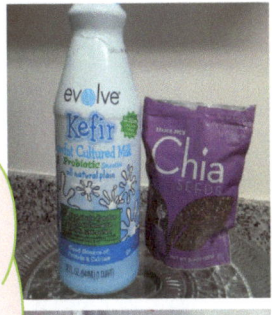
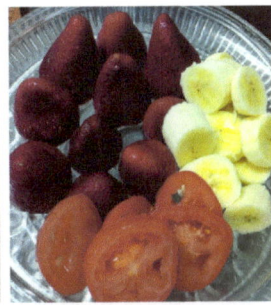

I am always so intrigued by this smoothie. It's tart and mildly sweet.

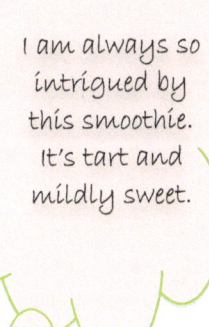
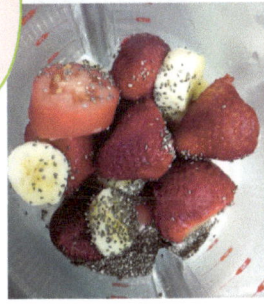
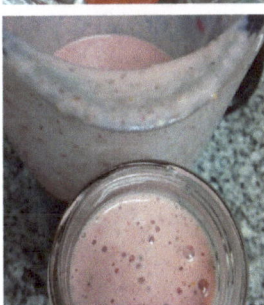

Notepad

Oatmeal Cookie

INGREDIENTS

1 cup Coconut Milk	1 Tbsp. Chia Flaxseed Blend	1 cup Oats soaked overnight	1 Tbsp. Honey	1 cup Spinach	Day 11
1 Banana	1 tsp. Cinnamon	1 Tbsp. Almond Butter	Place all ingredients in blender. Blend until desired consistency.		

Oatmeal Cookies transports me back to my childhood.

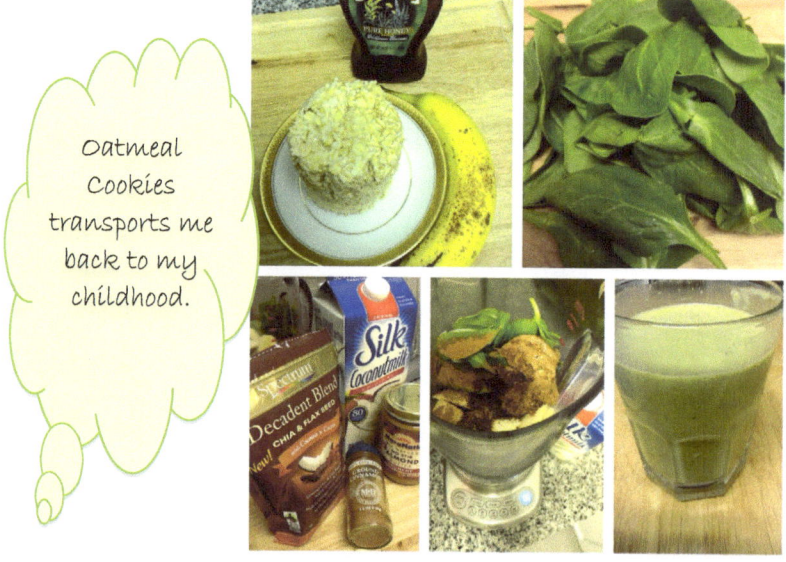

Notepad

Blueberry Pie

INGREDIENTS

1 cup Almond Milk	1 Tbsp. Almond Butter	1 cup Peaches	1 cup Blueberries	1 tsp. Cinnamon	**Day 12**
1 cup leftover Oats made with Almond, Chia Seeds, & Almond Milk			Place all ingredients in blender. Blend until desired consistency.		

I was introduced to blueberry pies later in life and I love them. I now enjoy that I can sip a Blueberry Pie.

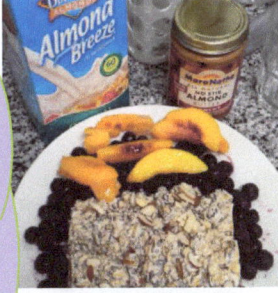

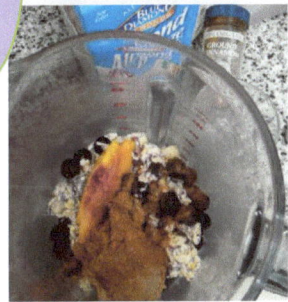

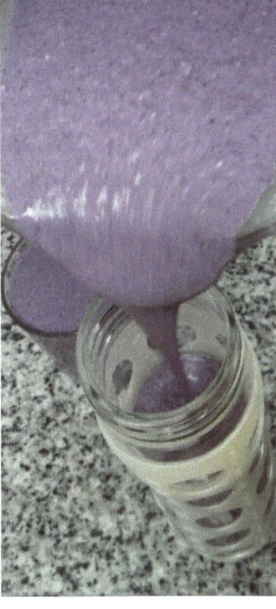

Notepad

PenandPaper.co.in

Nutty-Naughtiness

INGREDIENTS

1 cup Coconut Milk	1 Tbsp. Chia Flax Coconut Blend	1 Tbsp. Nutella	2 cups Strawberries	2 cups Cherries	**Day 13**
1 Celery stalk	Place all ingredients in blender. Blend until desired consistency.				

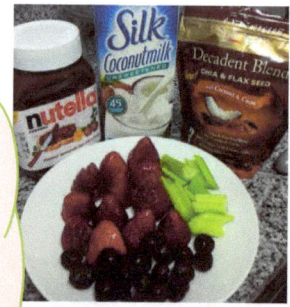

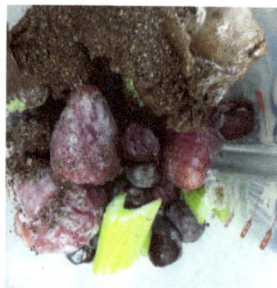

This smoothie is so intensely chocolaty. The Nutella brings all the ingredients together.

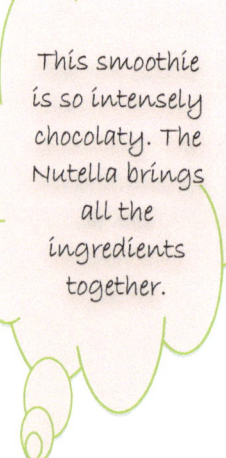

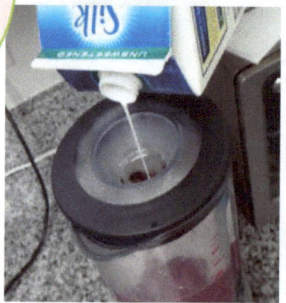

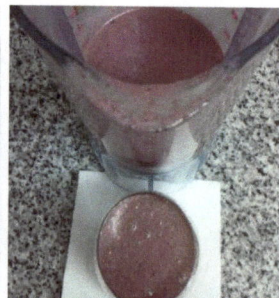

Notepad

PenandPaper.co.in

Summer Salad

INGREDIENTS

		½ cup grated Carrots	½ Lemon	2 cups Spinach	Day 14
1 cup Coconut Water	1 Tbsp. Hemp Seeds	1 Apple	1 Banana	1 Celery stalk	
3 Parsley sprigs		1 cup Mango	Place all ingredients in blender. Blend until desired consistency.		

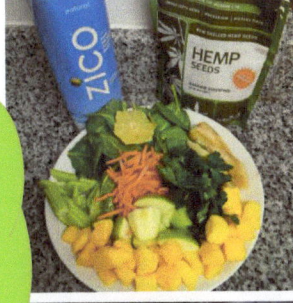
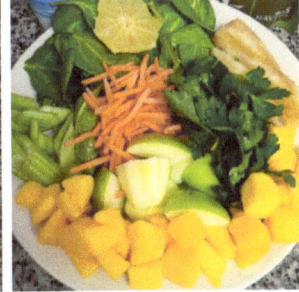

For me there is no denying that a well-orchestrated smoothie will leave you refreshingly satiated.

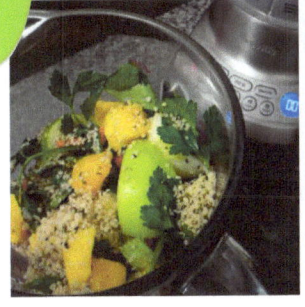
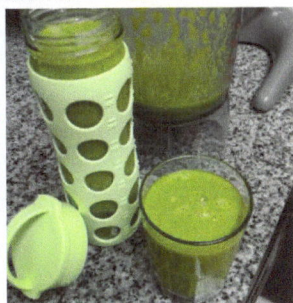

Notepad

Let's Get Freshical Freshical

INGREDIENTS

¼ cup Water	2 Grapefruits	2 Oranges	1 cup Mango	2 Tbsp. grated Ginger	Day 15
4–6 Mint leaves	1 Banana		Place all ingredients in blender. Blend until desired consistency.		

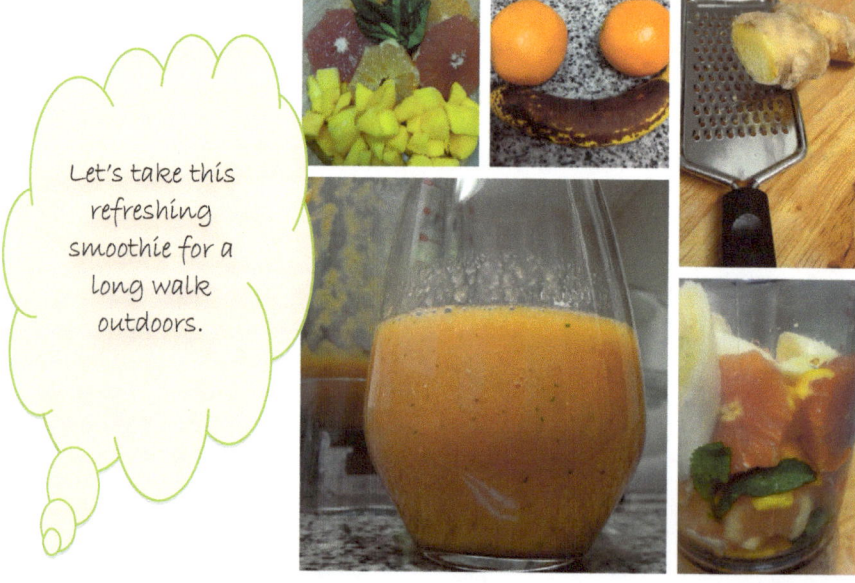

Let's take this refreshing smoothie for a long walk outdoors.

Notepad

An On-the-Go Kind of Day

INGREDIENTS

1 cup Almond Milk	½ cup cooked Oats	1 tsp. Cinnamon	3 dried Apricots	1 cup Blueberries	Day 16
2 large Kale leaves	1 Tbsp. Almond Butter	Place all ingredients in blender. Blend until desired consistency.			

The THINGS TO DO LIST is endless. Take your portable substance along for a boost of energy.

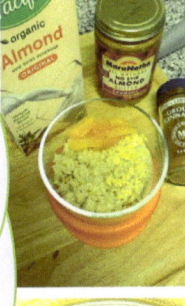
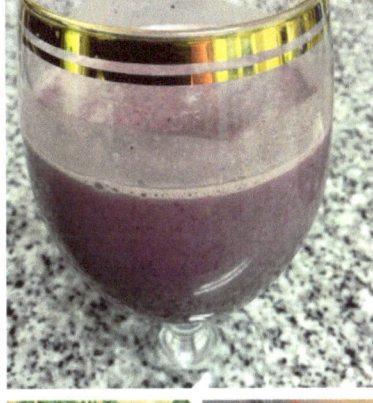

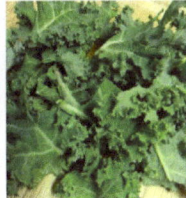
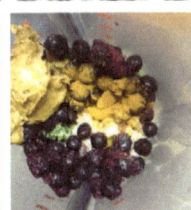

Notepad

Winter Be Gone

INGREDIENTS

1 cup Kefir	1 Tbsp. Flaxseed	1 cup Spinach	3 Kale leaves	1 cup Carrots	Day 17
1 Orange	1 Grapefruit	½ cup Peaches	1 cup Pineapple	Place all ingredients in blender. Blend until desired consistency.	

Banish the winter blahs with this wonderful reminder of spring.

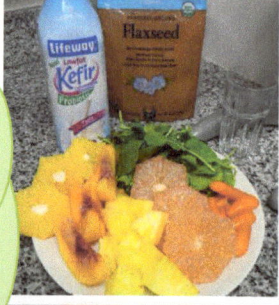

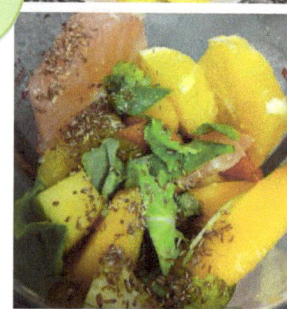

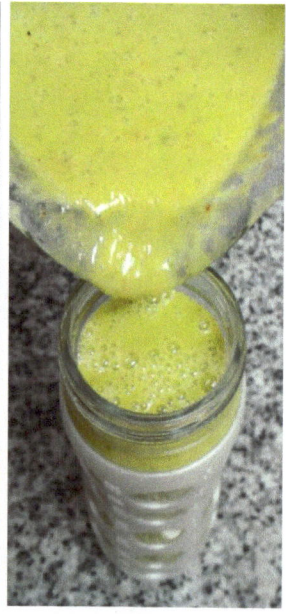

Notepad

Dessert on the Go

INGREDIENTS

1 cup Coconut Milk	1 Tbsp. Chia, Flax, Coconut Blend	1 Tbsp. Nutella	2 cups Strawberries	2 cups Peaches	Day 18
1 Banana	1 Celery stalk	Place all ingredients in blender. Blend until desired consistency.			

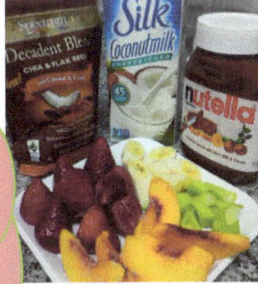

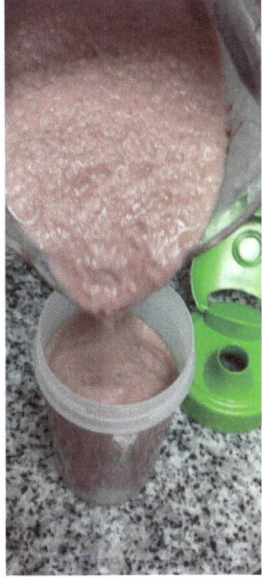

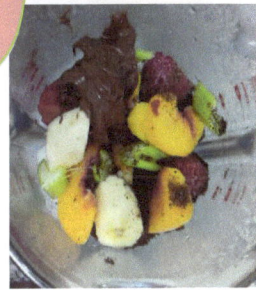

Using frozen and less Coconut Milk and fruit will turn this delight into a frozen "yogurt."

Notepad

Fresh and Clean

INGREDIENTS

1 cup fresh squeezed Orange Juice	1 Tbsp. Hemp Seeds	3 Kale leaves	1 Banana	1½ cups Strawberries	**Day 19**
1 Tbsp. grated Ginger	1 cup Mango	Place all ingredients in blender. Blend until desired consistency.			

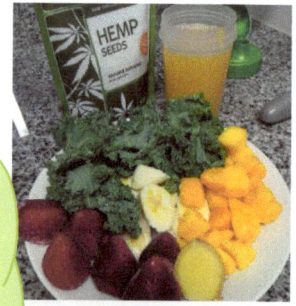
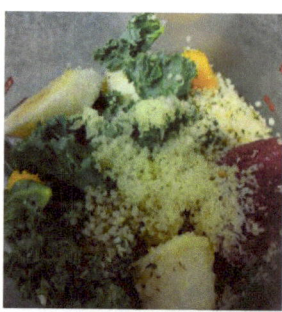
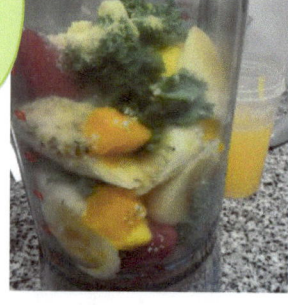
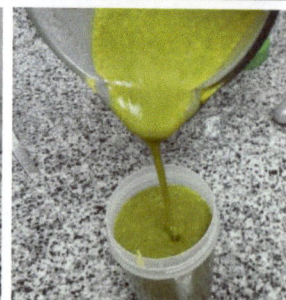

Sipping this smoothie makes me feel like I am doing something good for my tummy.

Notepad

Drink Your Nutrients

INGREDIENTS

1 cup Almond Milk	1 Tbsp. Chia Seeds	1 Tbsp. Almond Butter	3 Kale leaves	1 cup Blueberries	Day 20
½ Lemon	Zest of ½ Lemon	1 Banana	Place all ingredients in blender. Blend until desired consistency.		

This simple purple pleaser is wonderfully filling. I tend to have this around lunch time.

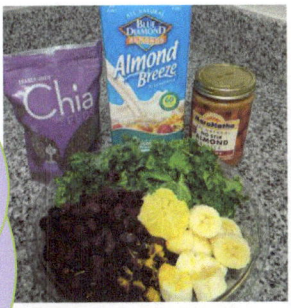

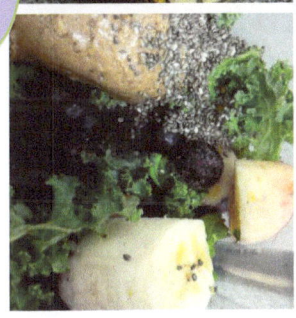

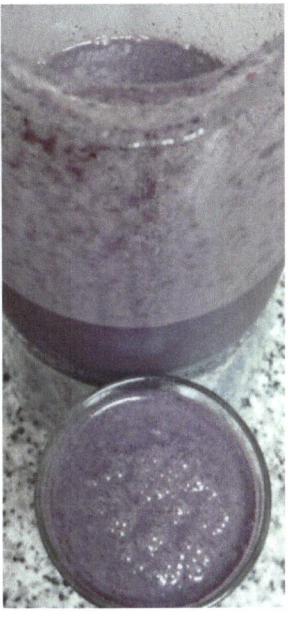

Notepad

Fruit Cocktail 2.0

INGREDIENTS

1 cup Kefir	1 Tbsp. Flaxseed	1 Grapefruit / 1 Orange	1 Lemon & Lemon zest	1 cup Mango	Day 21
½ cup Cherries	1 Tbsp. grated Ginger	1 Celery stalk	2 Parsley sprigs	2 cups Strawberries	Place all ingredients in blender. Blend until desired consistency.

Cheers!! To warmer weather, lighter food, and plenty of exercise.

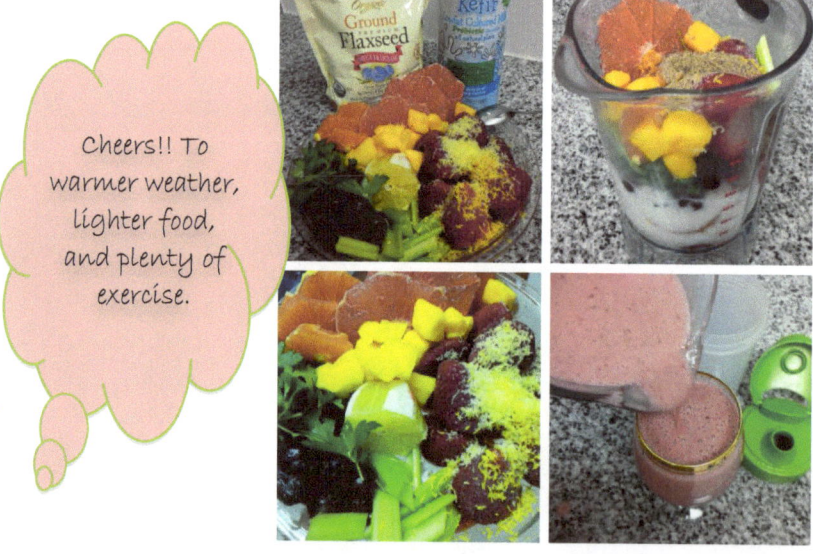

Notepad

Post Gym Punch

INGREDIENTS

1 cup Almond Milk	1 Tbsp. Chia Seeds	2 cups Spinach	1 cup Grapes	½ Lemon & zest	Day 22
2 Tbsp. Almond Butter	1 cup Peaches	1 cup Blueberries	Place all ingredients in blender. Blend until desired consistency.		

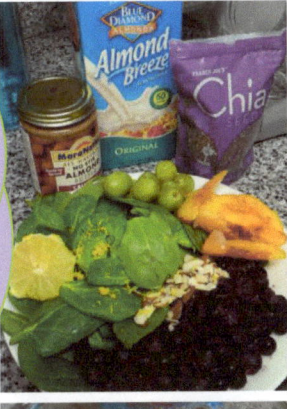

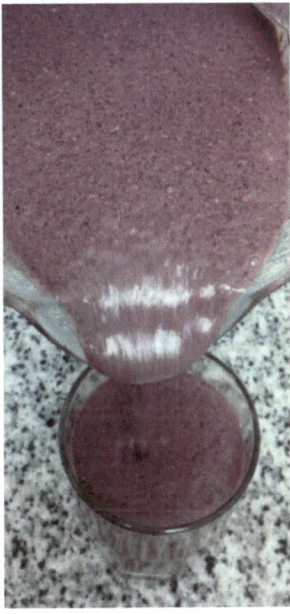

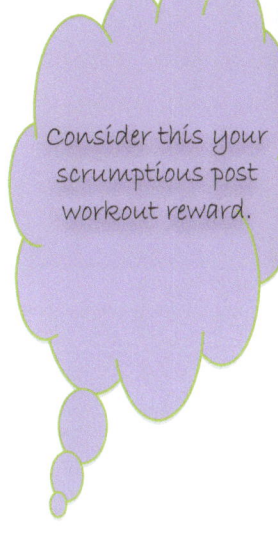

Consider this your scrumptious post workout reward.

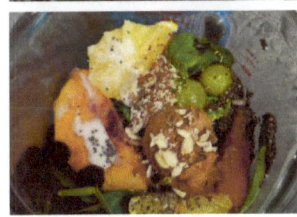

Notepad

Aloe-ha!

INGREDIENTS

1 Aloe leaf, split in half. Remove inner gel by scraping the gel with a spoon.	2 Oranges	3 Tbsp. grated Ginger	Day 23
½ cup Aloe Gel inner fillet	1 Grapefruit	2 cups Ice	
½ tsp. Cayenne Pepper	1 Lime	1 Tbsp. Turmeric	

Place all ingredients in blender. Blend until desired consistency.

I grew tired of buying factory-processed Aloe Gel/Juice...so I made my own. We shall call it Aloe Citrus Juice.

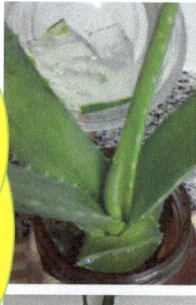
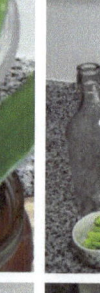
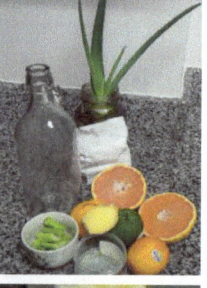
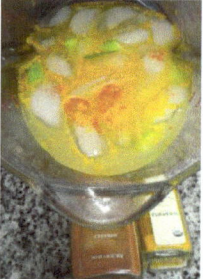
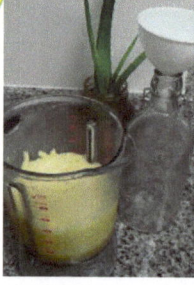
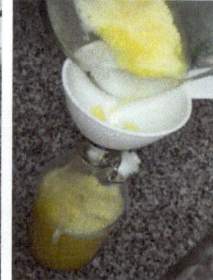
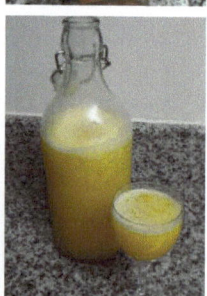

Notepad

The Kitchen Sink

INGREDIENTS

1 cup Coconut Water	1 Tbsp. Chia Seeds	1 Tbsp. Bee Pollen	1 Lemon	1 Celery stalk	1 Banana	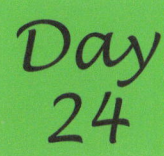 Day 24
1 Tbsp. Turmeric	1 cup Carrots	3 Kale leaves	1 cup Mango	1 Tbsp. grated Ginger		

Place all ingredients in blender. Blend until desired consistency.

For me there is no denying that one carefully orchestrated smoothie will leave you refreshingly satiated.

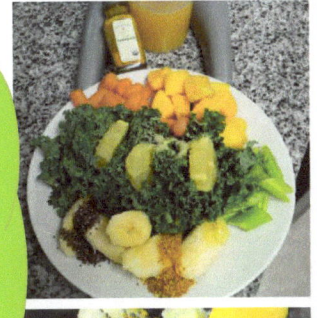
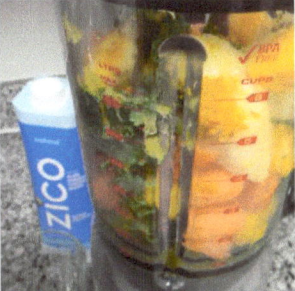
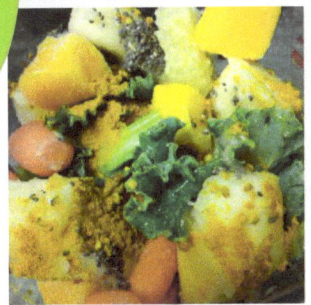
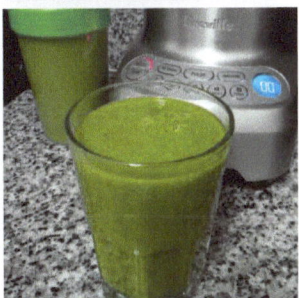

Notepad

Avo-Cherry-Berry

INGREDIENTS

1 cup Almond Milk	1 Tbsp. Chia, Flax, Coconut Blend	1 Tbsp. Almond Butter	1 cup Cherries	1 cup Strawberries	Day 25
1 Banana	1 Avocado	Place all ingredients in blender. Blend until desired consistency.			

There is no need to be pedestrian in your ingredient selection. Make your smoothies exciting.

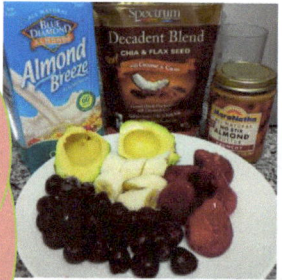
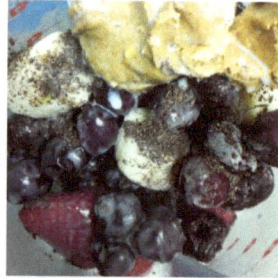
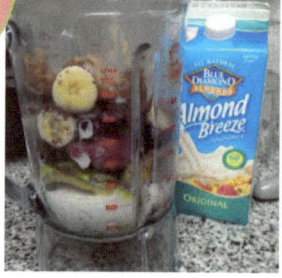
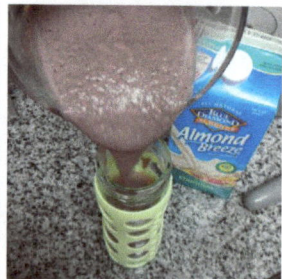

Notepad

Bee-ing Rejuvenated

INGREDIENTS

1 cup Coconut Water	1 Tbsp. Bee Pollen	1 Tbsp. grated Ginger	1 Grapefruit	1 cup Mango	Day 26
	2 cups Spinach	1 cup Pineapple			
1 cup Carrots	½ Lemon	1 Orange	Place all ingredients in blender. Blend until desired consistency.		

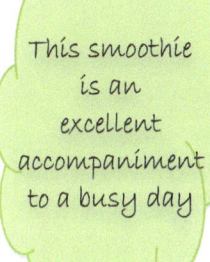

This smoothie is an excellent accompaniment to a busy day

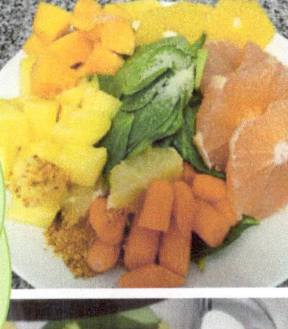

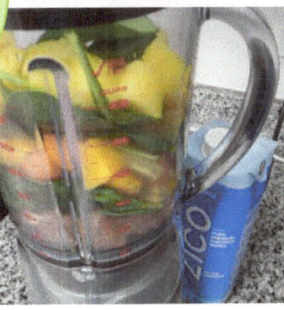

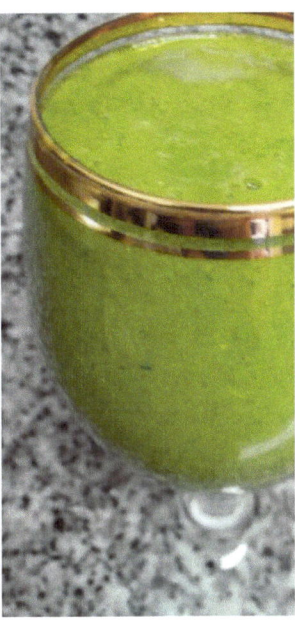

Notepad

Beet-It!

INGREDIENTS

1 cup Almond Milk	1 Tbsp. Flaxseed	1 steamed Red Beet	1 cup Pineapple	1 Banana	**Day 27**
½ Lemon	2 cups Strawberries	Place all ingredients in blender. Blend until desired consistency.			

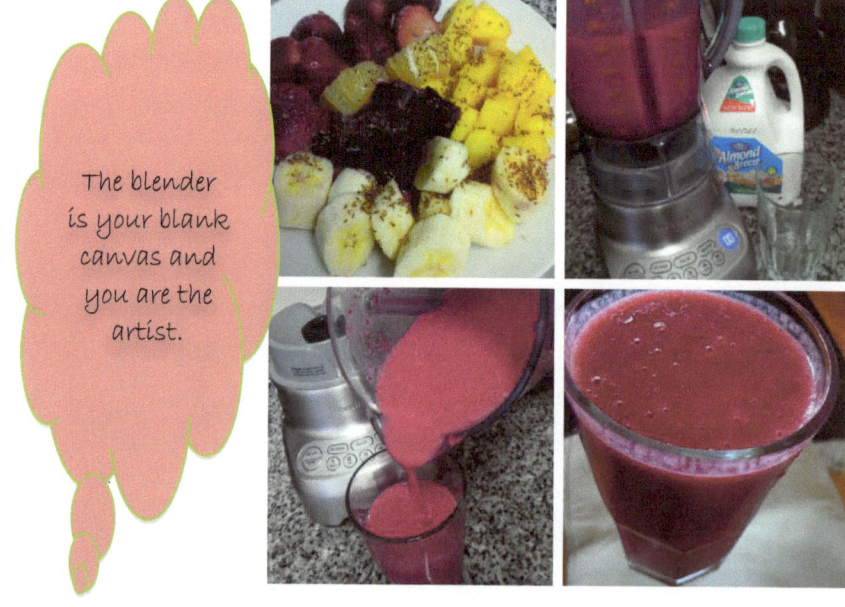

The blender is your blank canvas and you are the artist.

Notepad

Piña-Kale-Ada

INGREDIENTS

1 cup Coconut Milk	1 Tbsp. Flaxseed	3 Kale leaves	1 cup Pineapple	1 cup Mango	1 Banana	Day 28
½ cup Peaches	2 Celery stalks	Place all ingredients in blender. Blend until desired consistency.				

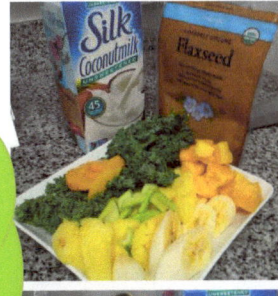

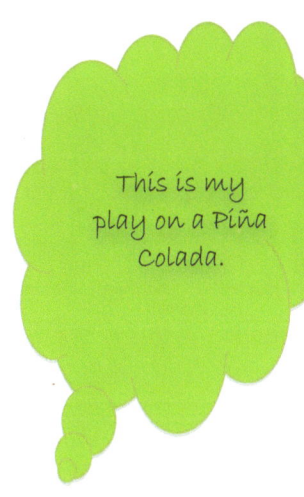

This is my play on a Piña Colada.

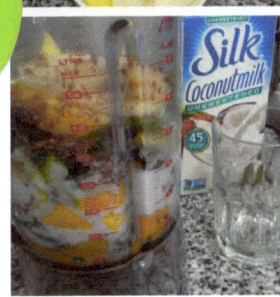

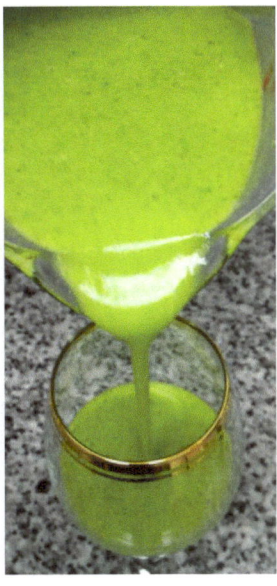

Notepad

3 Meals in 1, done!

INGREDIENTS

1 cup Almond Milk	1 Tbsp. Nutella	1 cup Strawberries	1 cup leftover Oats made with Almond, Chia Seeds, Raisins, & Almond Milk	Day 29
Place all ingredients in blender. Blend until desired consistency.				

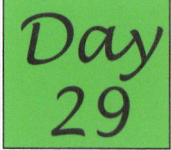

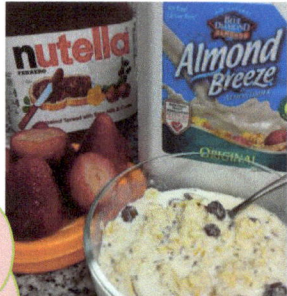

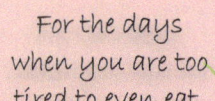

For the days when you are too tired to even eat.

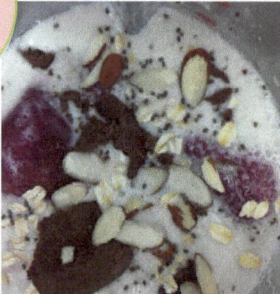

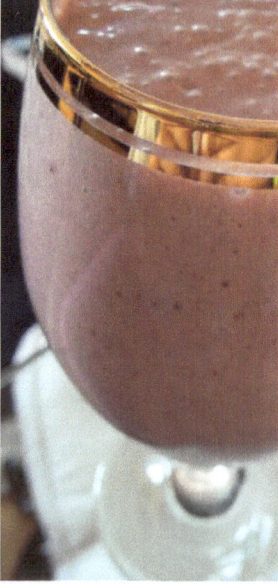

Notepad

Exotic Probiotic

INGREDIENTS

1 cup Kefir	1 Tbsp. Bee Pollen	2 cups Watermelon	1 cup Mango	1 Banana	2 Celery stalks	Day 30
2 cups Spinach	½ Lemon	Place all ingredients in blender. Blend until desired consistency.				

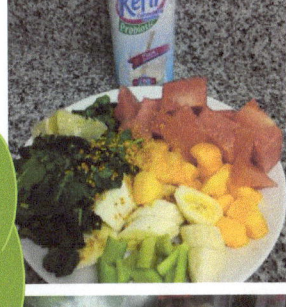

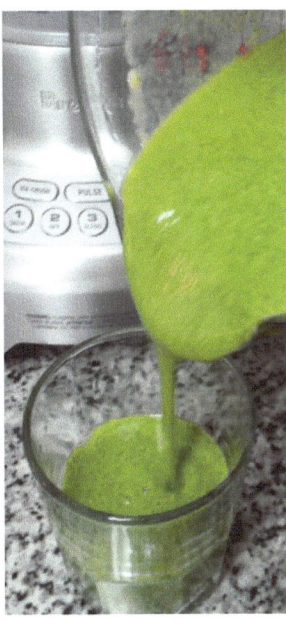

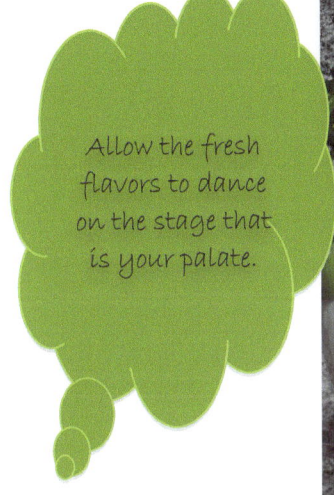

Allow the fresh flavors to dance on the stage that is your palate.

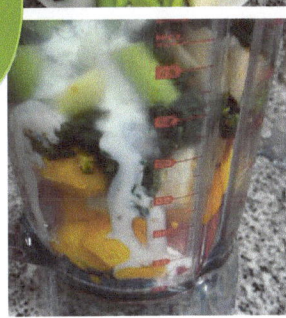

Notepad

The Almond Brothers

INGREDIENTS

1 cup Almond Milk	1 Tbsp. Chia Seeds	1 Tbsp. Almond Butter	2 cups Blueberries	1 Banana	Day 31
¼ cup Almonds	2 cups Mango	Place all ingredients in blender. Blend until desired consistency.			

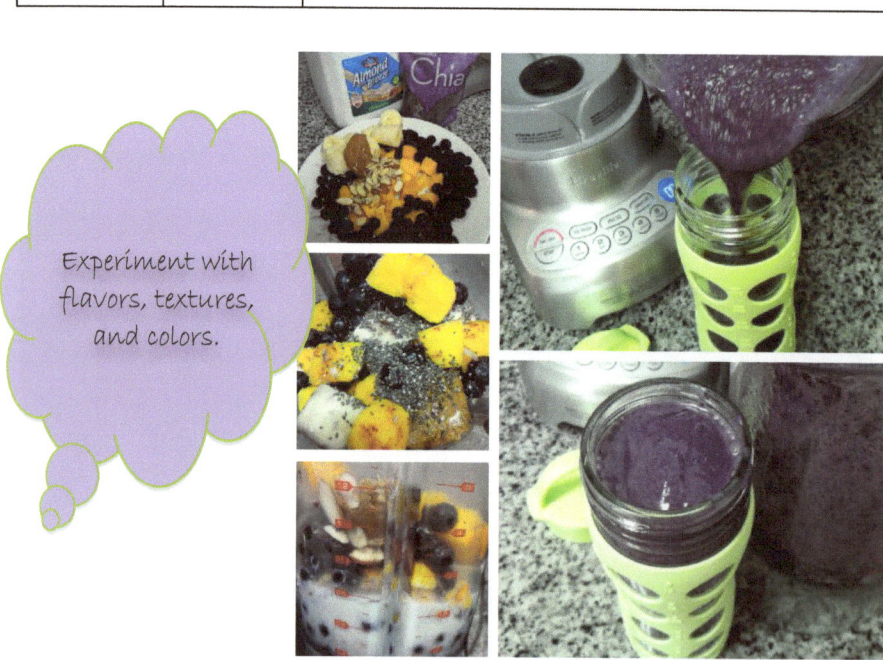

Experiment with flavors, textures, and colors.

Notepad

…and in closing. Allow me to thank you one more time.

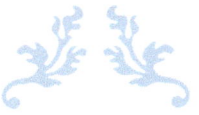

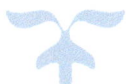

During this journey into smoothie creations, I have come to realize that we overfeed ourselves because we have this need to literally feel full. This feeling-full experience is what's packing on the pounds/kilos. We tend to overfeed ourselves for fear of starvation, I guess, or the "I don't want to be hungry later" line. We need to resist the urge to clean the plate. When our tummy and brain tell us to STOP EATING, YOU ARE FULL!!!

The rules are simple:

BURN MORE CALORIES THAN YOU CONSUME
Add more fruits and vegetables to your diet
Try to go two days without meat
Results will come if you persevere
Make good food choices
Everything in moderation

Results are reflected when you have a balanced diet and regular exercise.

Thank you for taking the time to read my book. I do so hope you've enjoyed this blended journey of interesting palate-pleasing smoothies.

I am so pleased with myself for undertaking this personal challenge of cleansing my body on a cellular level. I lost weight and gained the trust within myself to see this journey through.

PS: No animals were harmed in the making of this book.

—*xox*—
Cecelia

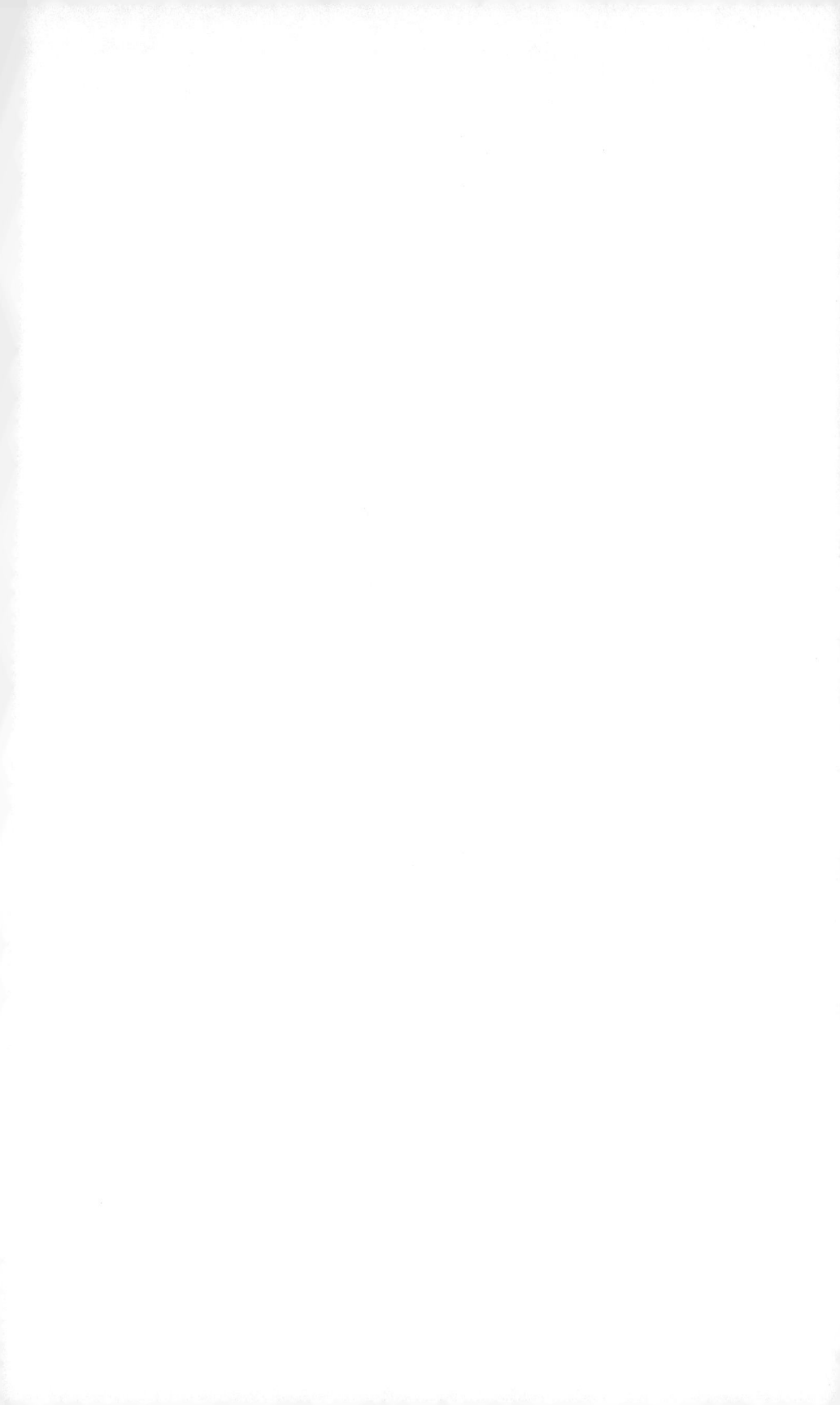

www.ingramcontent.com/pod-product-compliance
Lightning Source LLC
Chambersburg PA
CBHW050835290526
45792CB00001B/404